Chiari for Kids

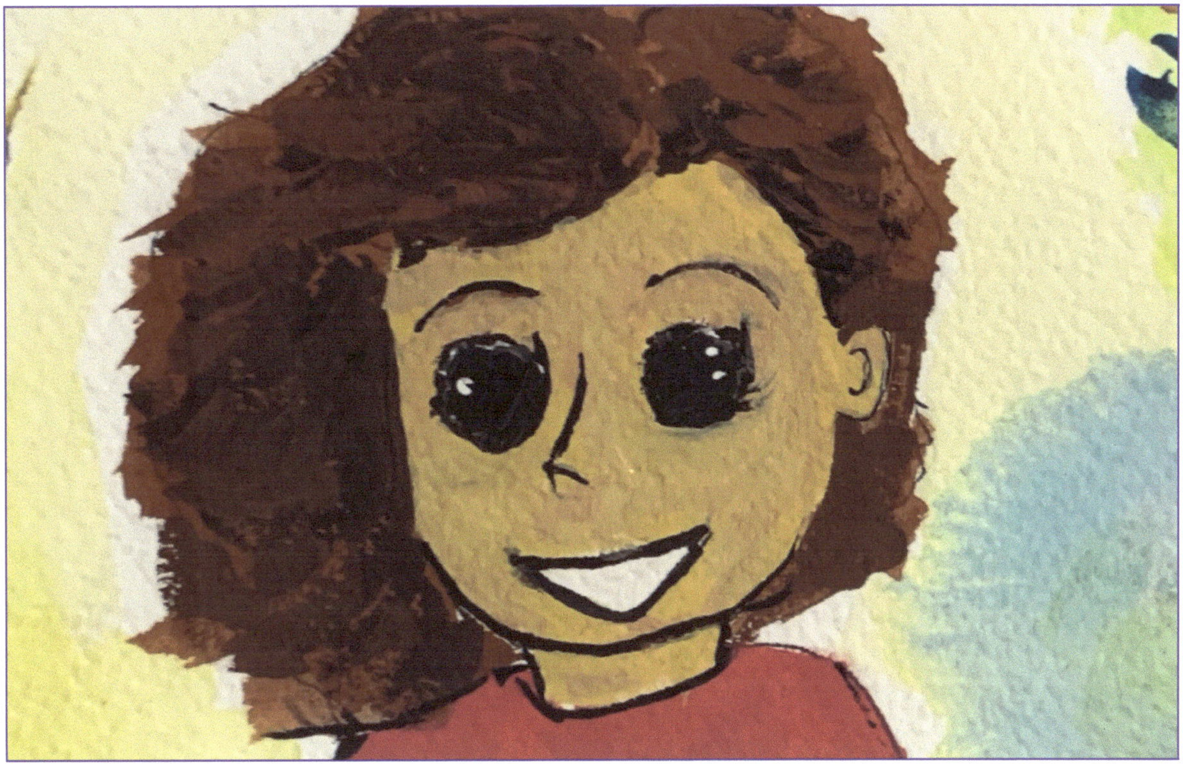

By Tiffany Crespo

HI! MY NAME IS TIFFANY, BUT MY FRIENDS CALL ME "TIFF".

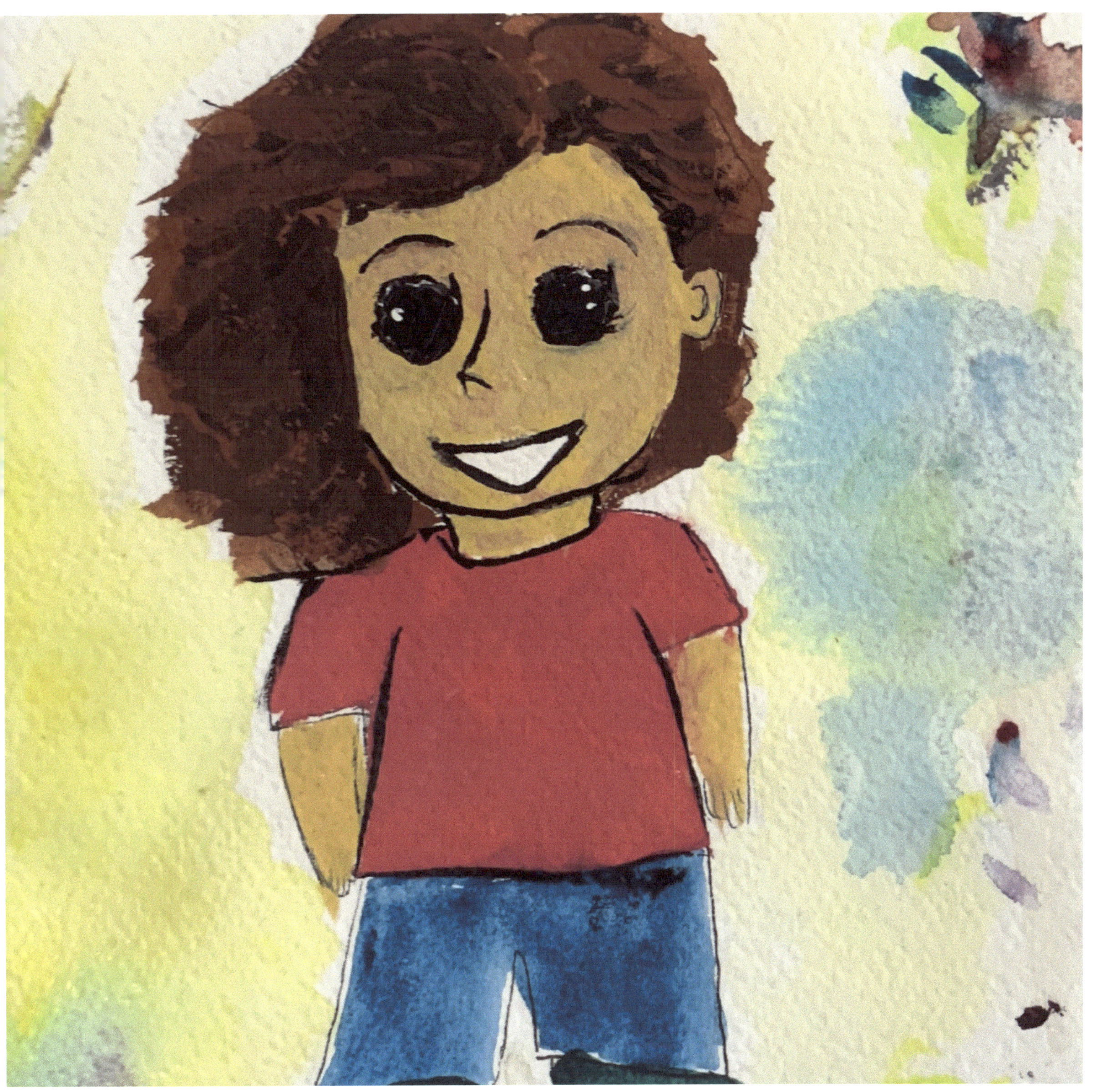

I GUESS YOU COULD SAY THAT
I HAVE A BIG BRAIN.

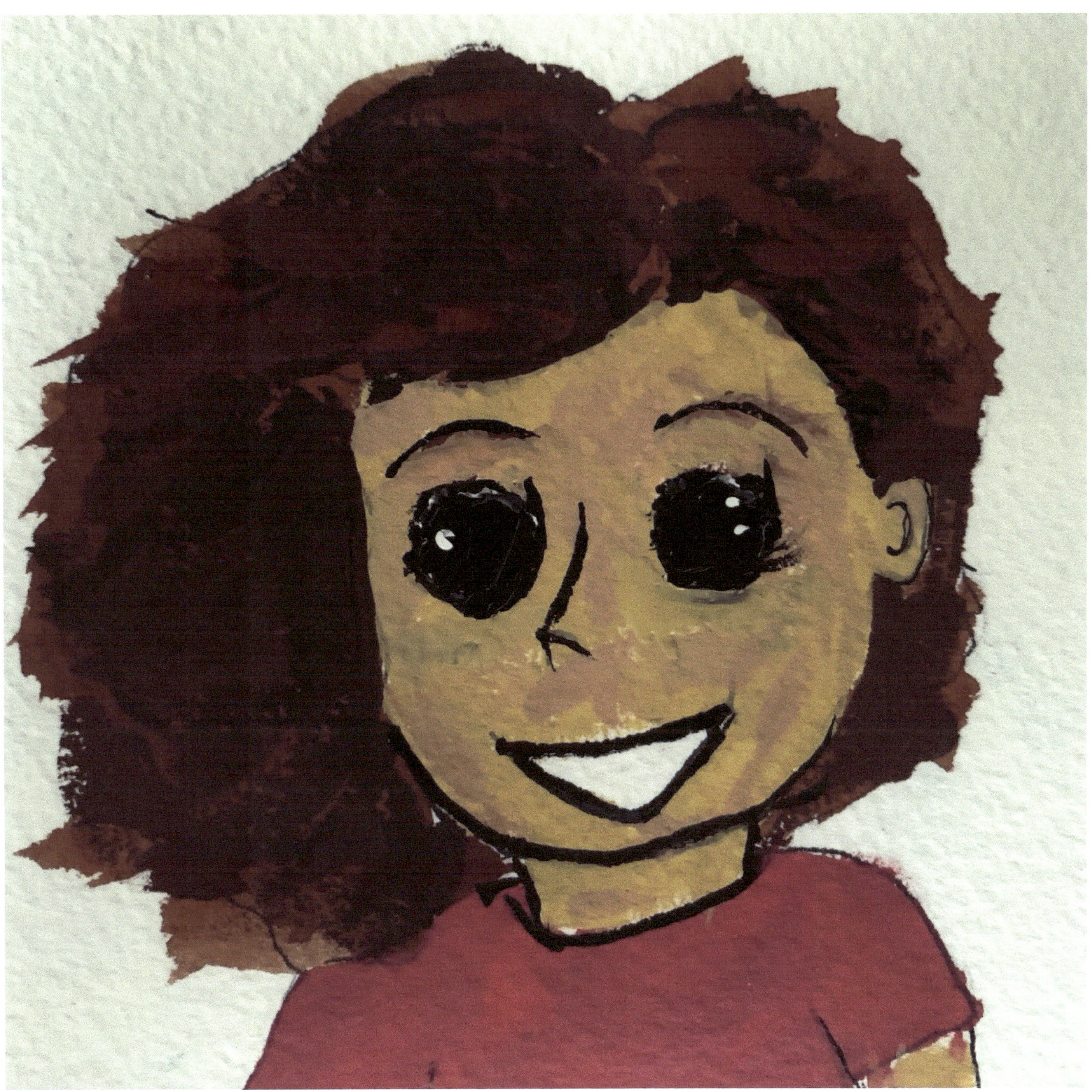

MY DAD SAYS IT'S WHAT MAKES ME SO SMART BUT HE'S MY DAD AND HAS TO SAY THAT.

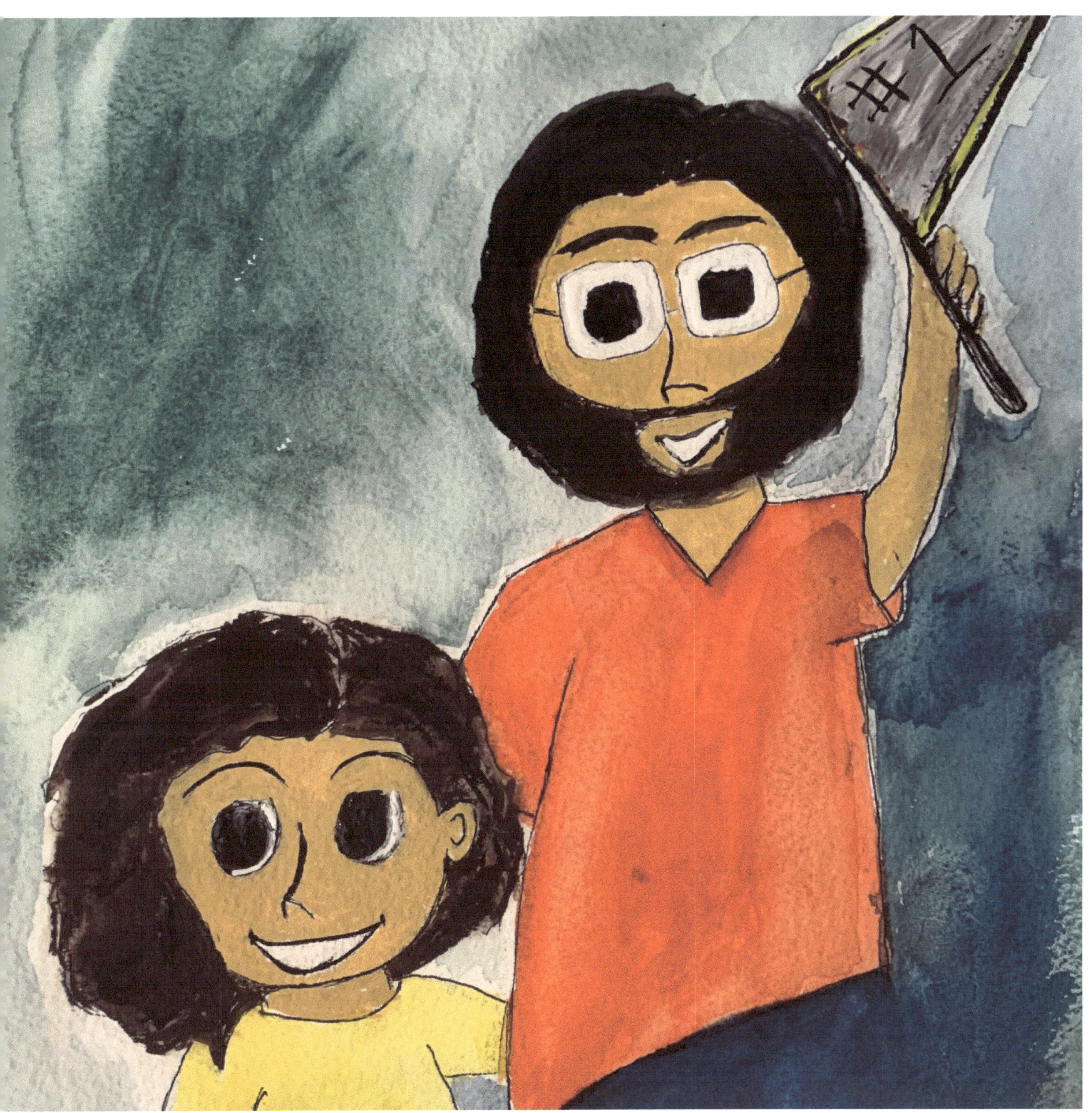
#1

MY DOCTOR SAYS I'M BRAVE
BECAUSE OF IT
BUT SHE'S REALLY NICE
AND LIKES TO
MAKE ME SMILE.

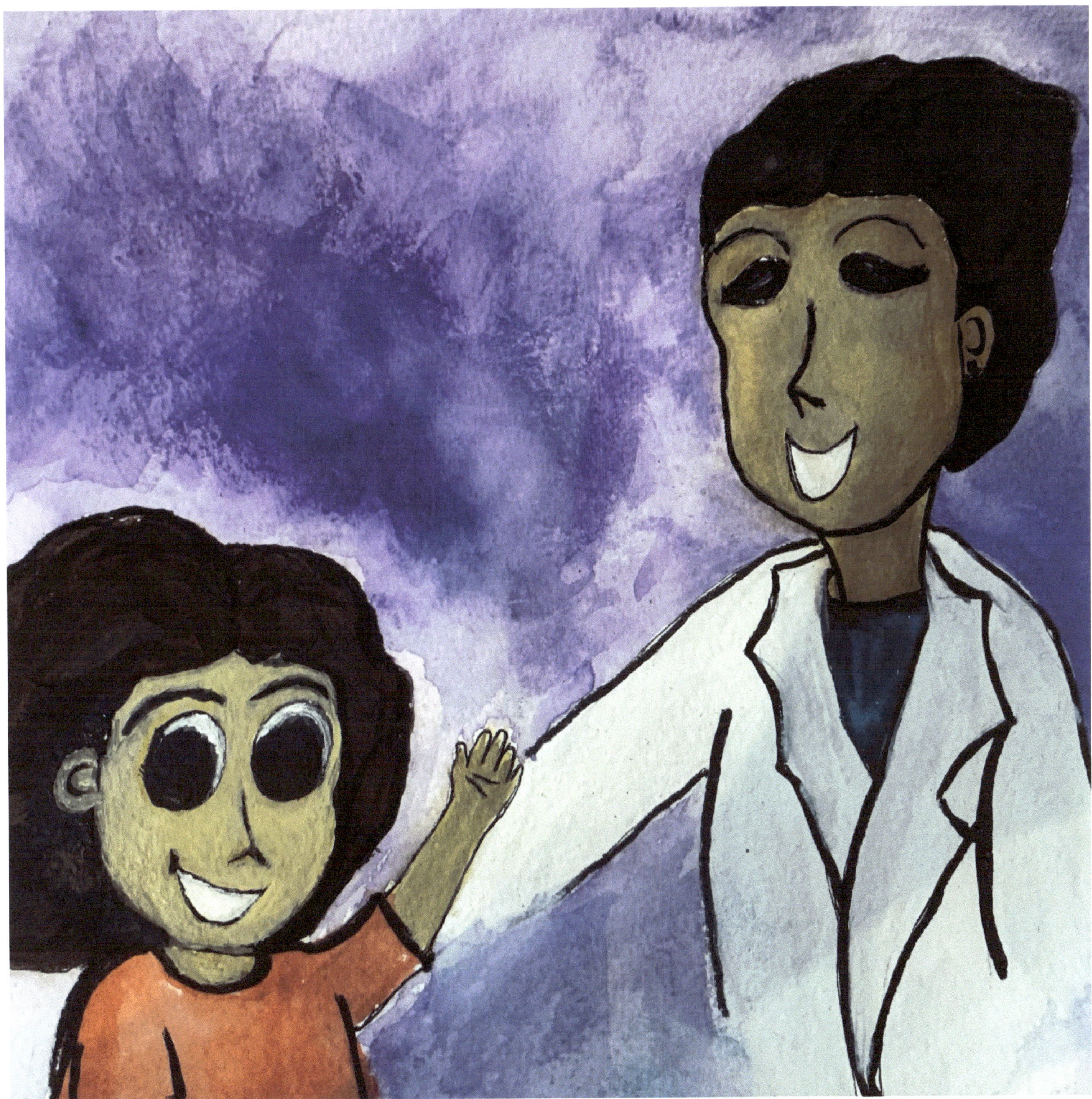

I WAS BORN WITH AN ARNOLD CHIARI MALFORMATION.

IT'S A BIG NAME SO
I CALL IT "CHIARI".

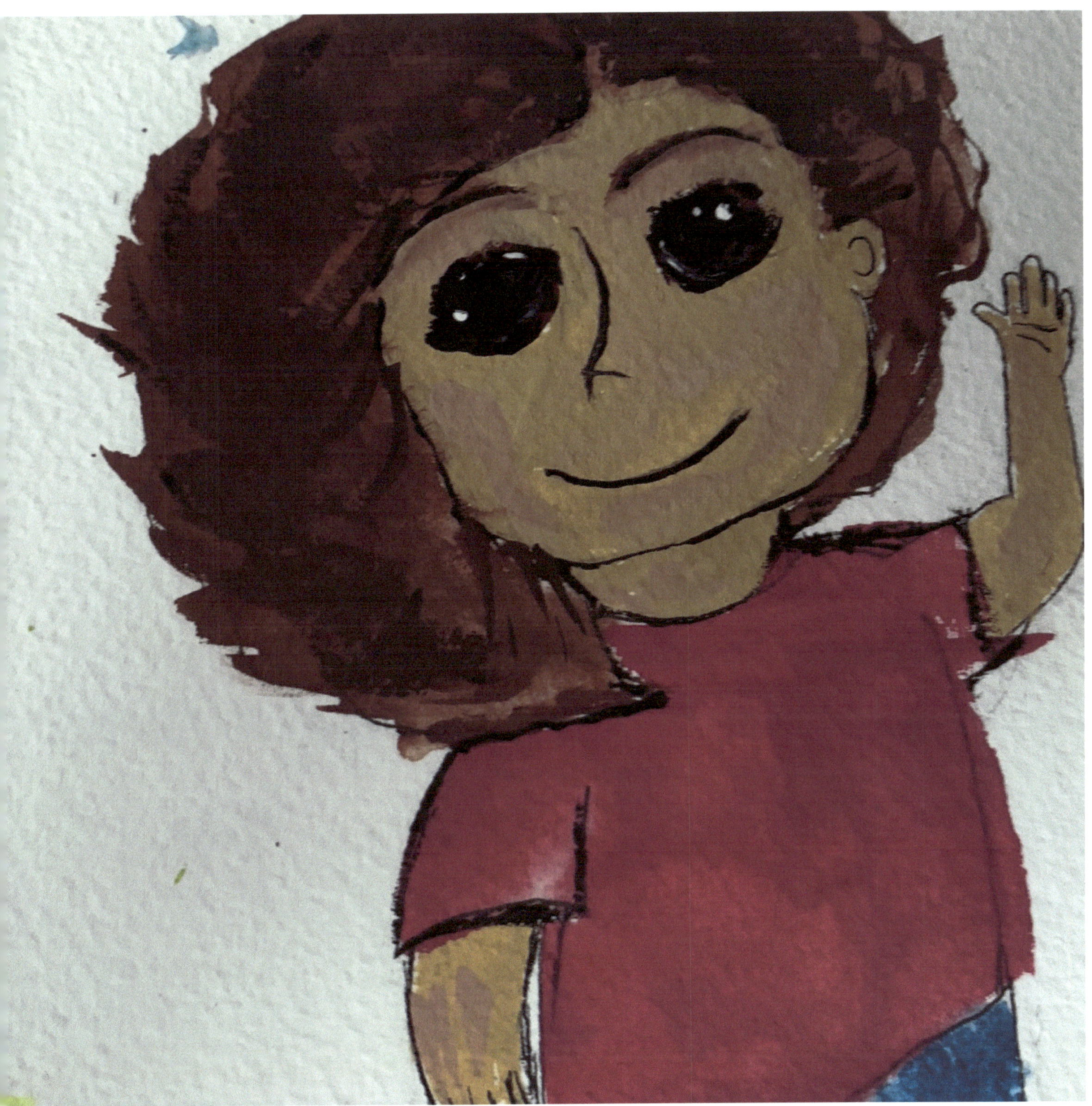

CHIARI IS WHEN YOUR BRAIN TISSUE
EXTENDS INTO
YOUR SPINAL CANAL.

THIS CAN CAUSE PRESSURE ON BOTH
YOUR BRAIN AND THE NERVES IN YOUR
SPINE.

SYMPTOMS CAN BE MILD
TO SEVERE.

YOU CAN SAY IT LIKE THIS...

"KEY- R- E"

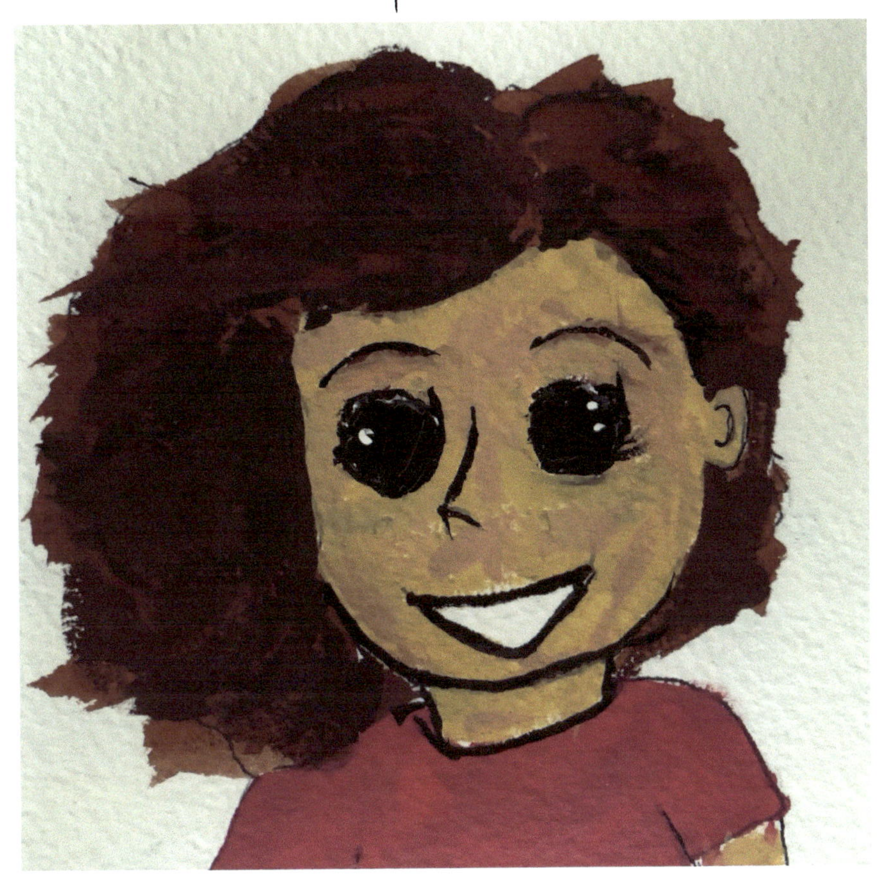

COMMON SYMPTOMS ARE INTENSE PRESSURE HEADACHES AND DIZZINESS.

SOMETIMES YOU MAY HAVE BALANCE DIFFICULTIES AND MAY HAVE PROBLEMS WALKING OR EVEN TALKING.

OFTEN SURGERY IS NEEDED AND SOME MAY EVEN REQUIRE MORE THAN ONE TO FEEL BETTER.

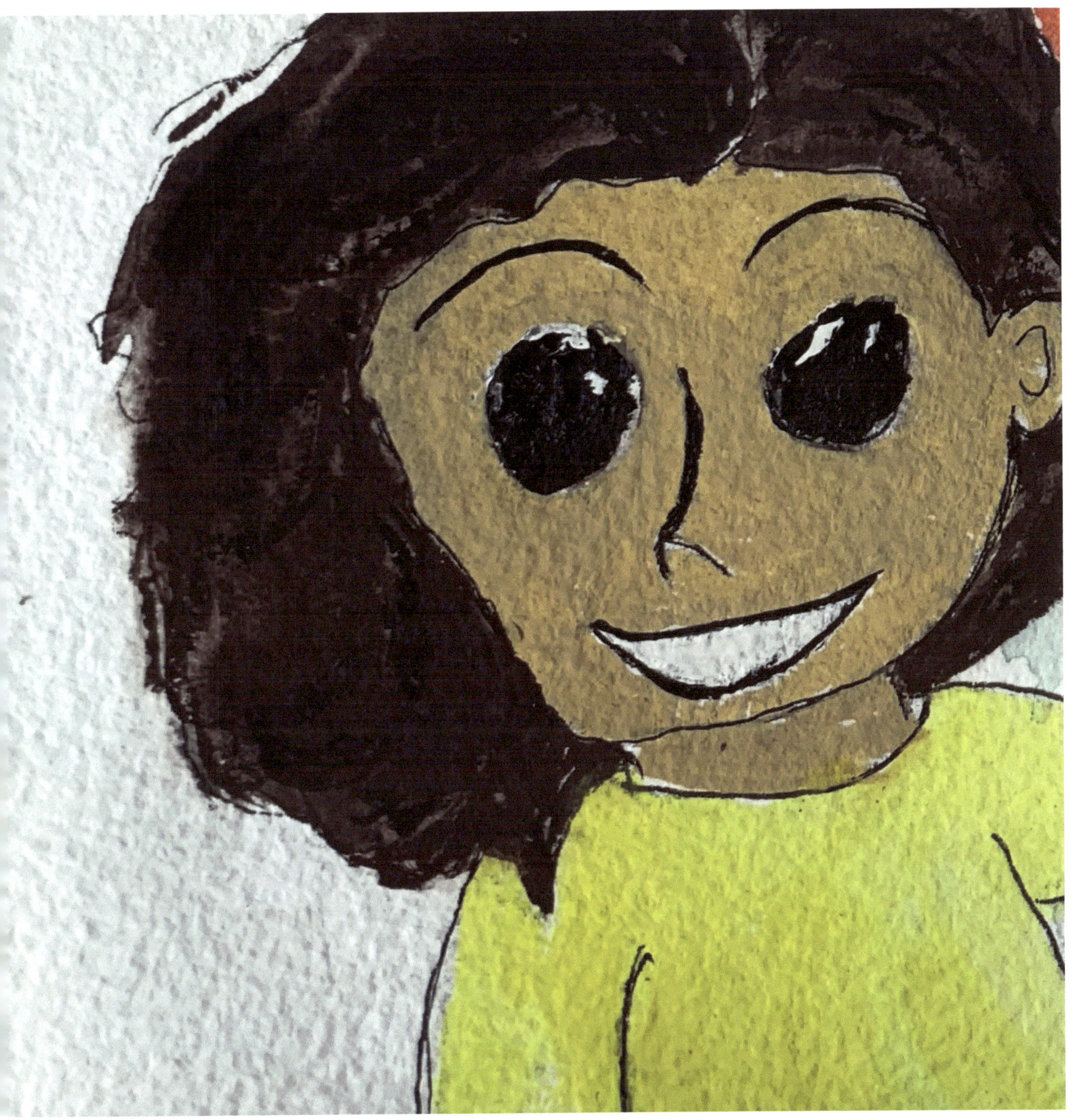

BEING TOLD I WOULD NEED SURGERY WAS REALLY SCARY.

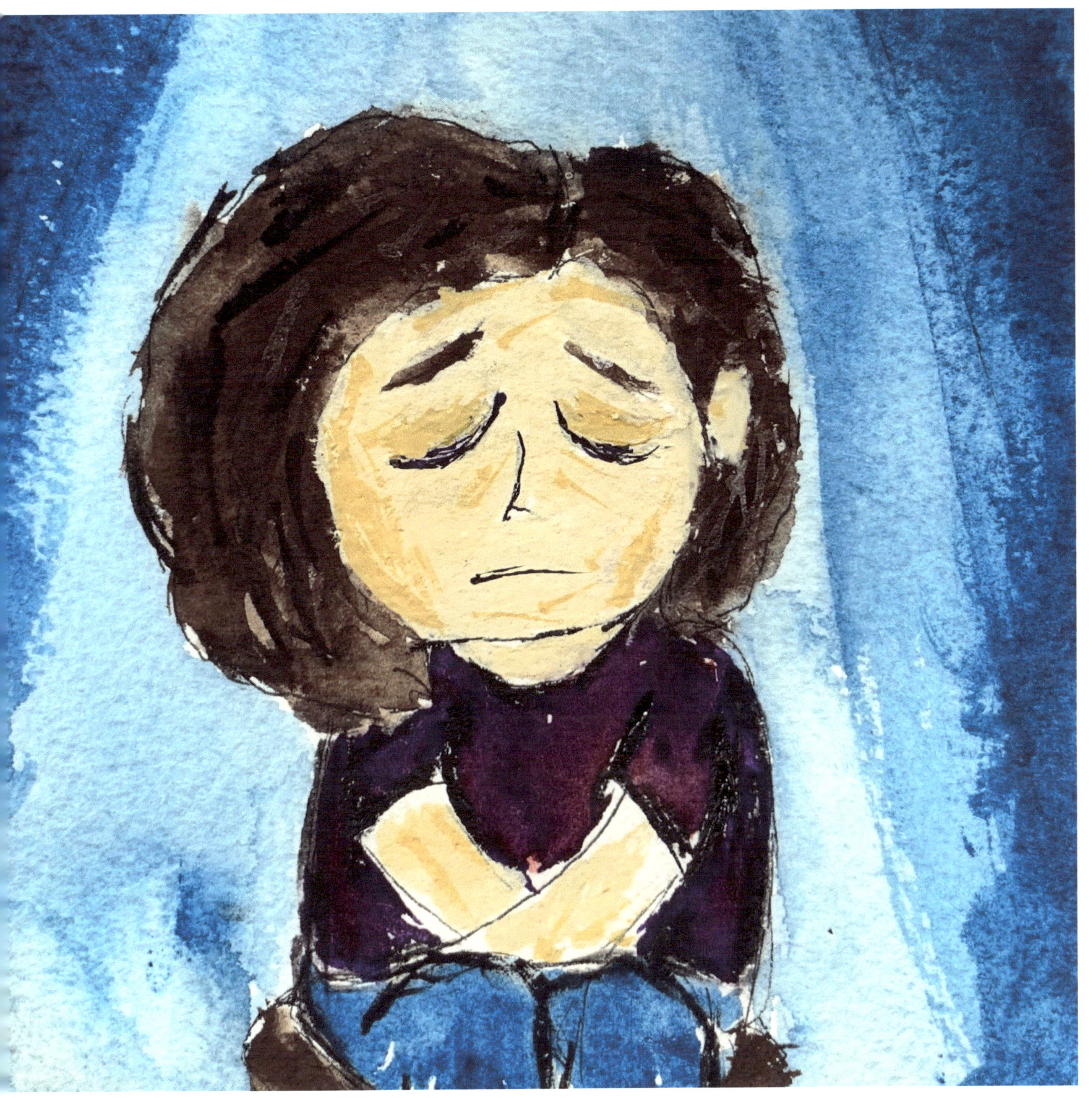

IT'S OKAY

TO BE AFRAID!

SURGERY WENT WELL AND I NOW
EVEN HAVE A COOL SCAR!
SOME OF US WHO GET
SURGERY CALL OURSELVES
"ZIPPERHEADS".
IT'S LIKE A CLUB AND I'M A MEMBER.

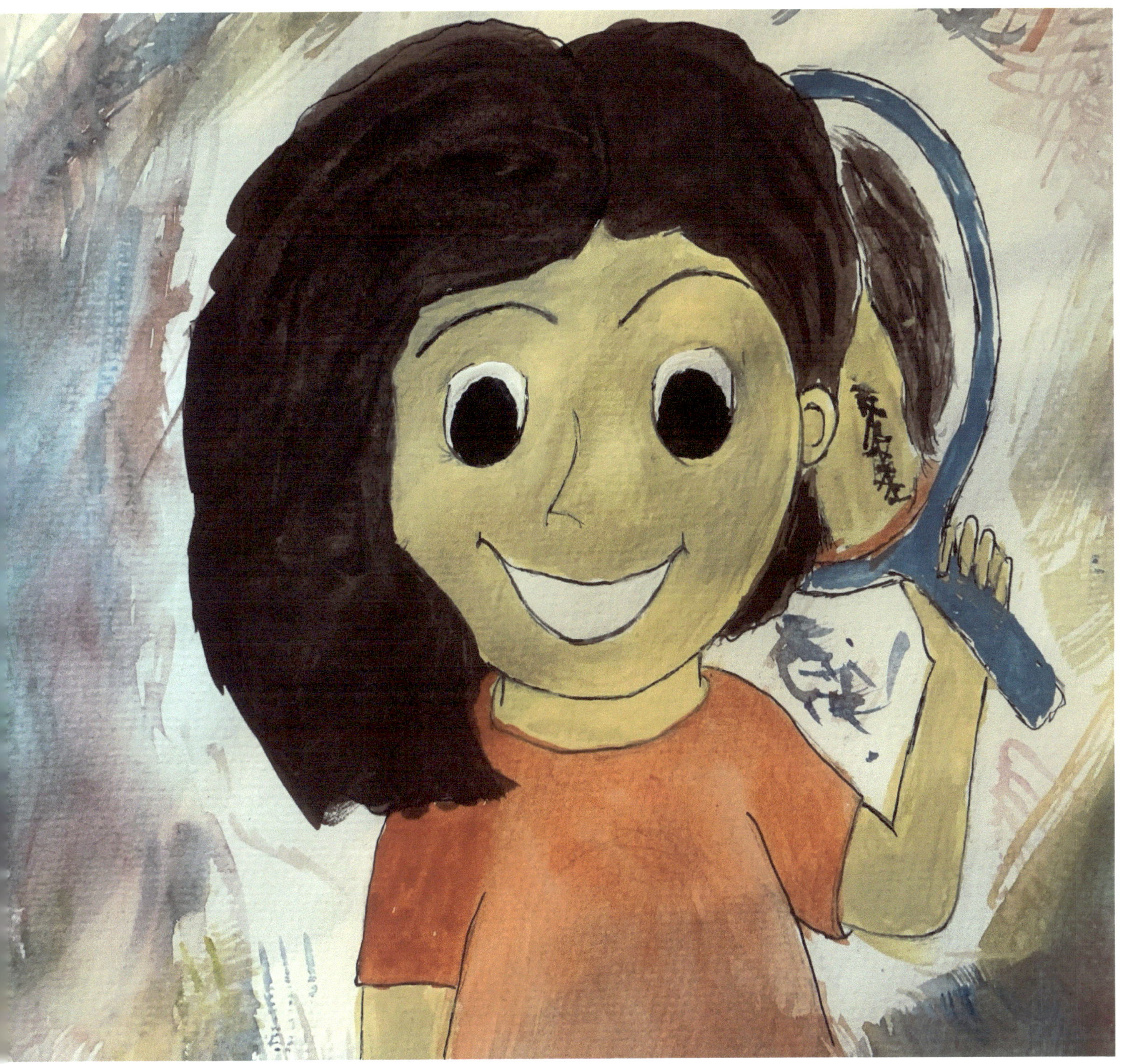

CHIARI COMES IN MANY SHAPES AND SIZES.

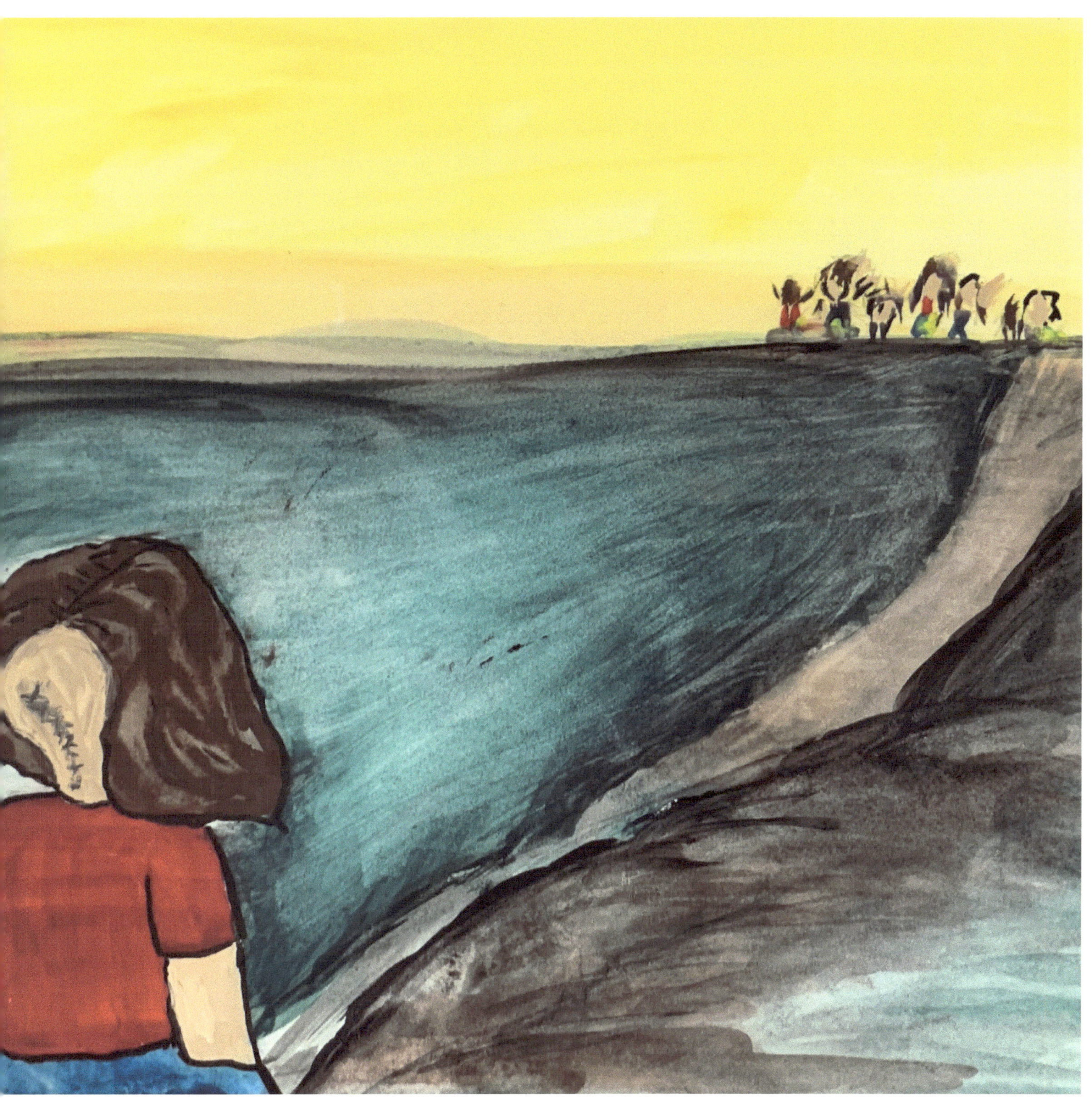

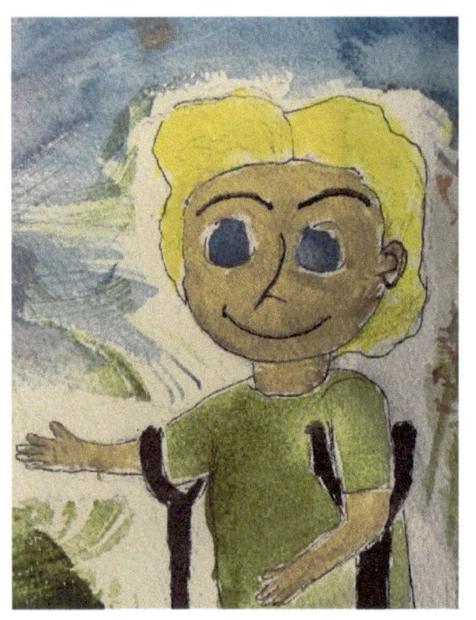

THIS IS EZRA. HE HAS CHIARI AND HAS HAD 2 SURGERIES TO HELP RELIEVE THE PRESSURE IN HIS HEAD. HE ALSO HAS A CONDITION CALLED SYRINGOMYELIA. THIS IS A DISORDER IN WHICH FLUID FILLED CYSTS (ALSO CALLED SYRINX) FORM IN THE SPINAL CORD.

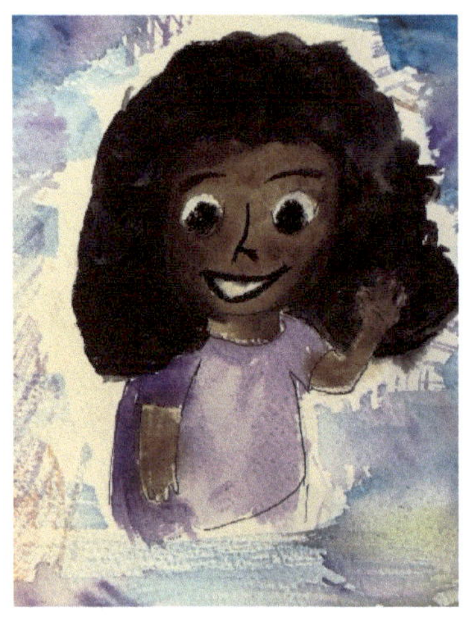

THIS IS AMY. SHE HAS CHIARI BUT CANNOT HAVE DECOMPRESSION SURGERY. IN ADDITION TO CHIARI, AMY ALSO HAS TRANSVERSE SINUS STENOSIS. THIS CAUSES HER TO EXPERIENCE ADDITIONAL DIZZINESS AND PRESSURE. HER DOCTORS ARE LOOKING AT OTHER OPTIONS TO HELP SUCH AS A SHUNT OR STENT.

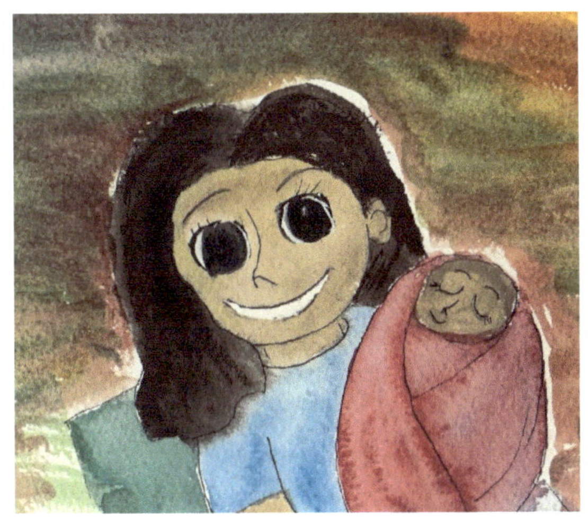

KIMBERLY AND HER DAUGHTER RACHEL WERE BOTH BORN WITH CHIARI MALFORMATIONS. KIMBERLY'S SYMPTOMS ARE MILD AND SHE HAS NEVER NEEDED SURGERY. RACHEL HAS ALREADY DISPLAYED SIGNS AND SYMPTOMS. SHE MAY REQUIRE SURGERY LATER AS A TODDLER.

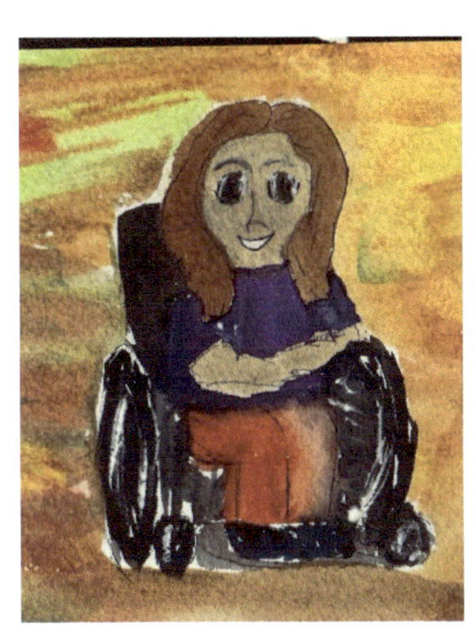

MANY WHO HAVE CHIARI HAVE SECONDARY CONDITIONS LIKE SPINA BIFIDA. THIS IS THE CASE FOR CARRIE.
CARRIE HAS HAD SEVERAL SURGERIES TO IMPROVE HER QUALITY OF LIFE.

EVEN THOUGH HAVING CHIARI CAN
SOMETIMES FEEL LONELY
REMEMBER,
THERE ARE OTHERS OUT THERE WHO
UNDERSTAND WHAT YOU ARE
EXPERIENCING.

TOGETHER WE CAN TEACH THE WORLD ABOUT CHIARI.

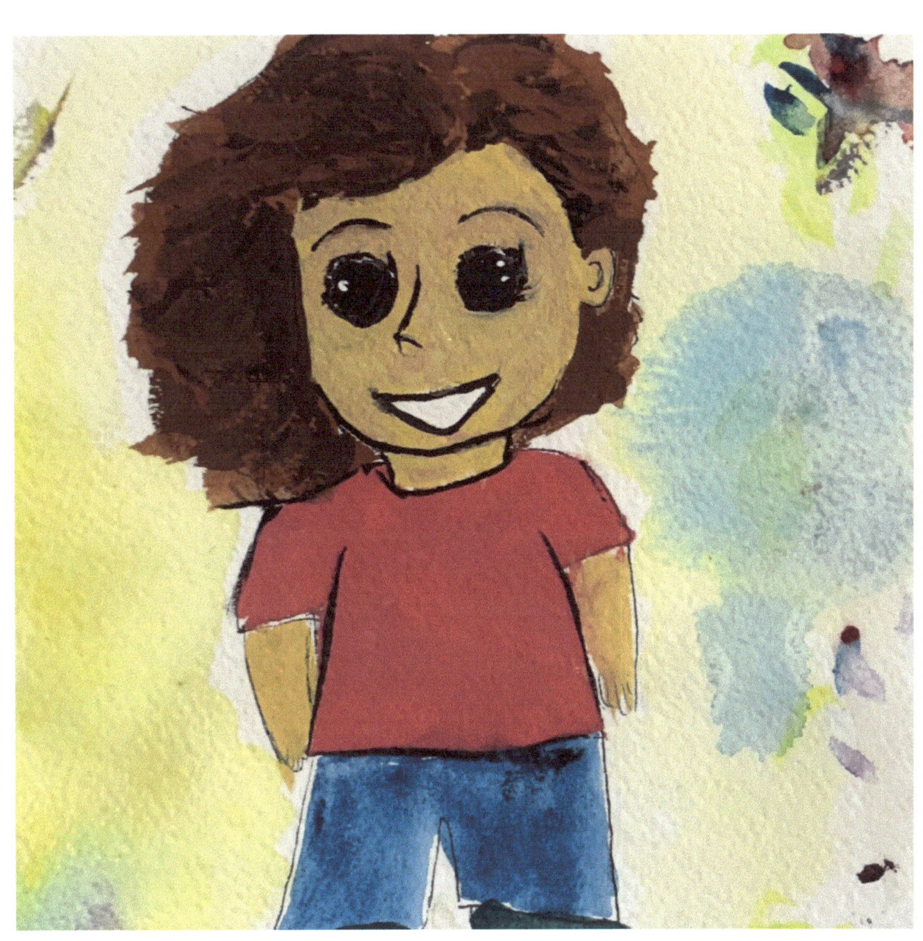

Chiari Resources

Johns Hopkins Medicine

https://www.hopkinsmedicine.org/health/
conditions-and-diseases/
chiari-malformation

Conquer Chiari

www.conquerchiari.org

National institute of Neurological
Disorders and Stroke

www.ninds.nih.gov

American Syringomyelia and Chiari Alliance project

www.ASAP.org

About the Author

Tiffany Crespo was diagnosed with Chiari in 2020
at the age of 38.
After years of discomfort and pain, an MRI ordered by her doctor revealed the malformation.

Tiffany traveled from Florida to Maryland
and had decompression surgery by
Dr. Judy Huang of Johns Hopkins University.

On July 28, 2020, Tiffany became a proud "Zipperhead".
Tiffany is also a proud mom to two boys and is just
"happy to be here".

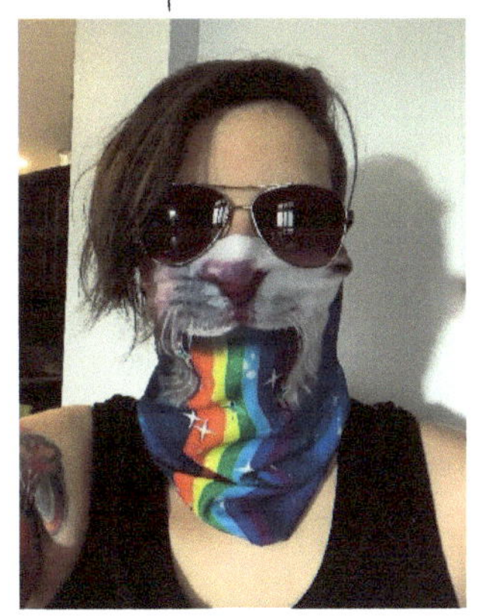

www.ingramcontent.com/pod-product-compliance
Ingram Content Group UK Ltd.
Pitfield, Milton Keynes, MK11 3LW, UK
UKHW060114300726
14090UKWH00002B/189

9798501111615